All Natural Soap

Making Recipes

Easy Soap Making Book to Make for

You and Your Loved Ones!

Table of Contents

Introduction

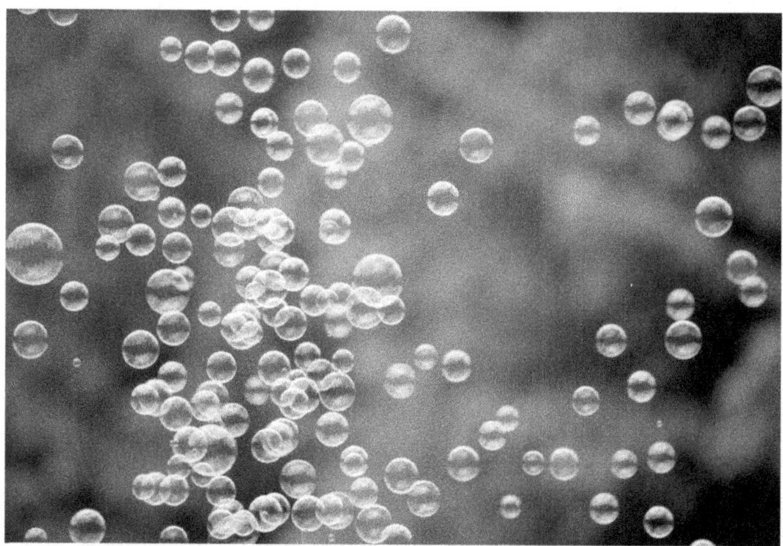

Thank you for getting a copy of this recipe book! I am glad that you have chosen the path to giving you skin a beautiful and glowing lift with homemade soaps.

Before we go into the soap recipes proper, it is imperative that I once again reiterate why you need to boycott store bought soaps and stick to the ones you make in your home.

First off, you are sure that there is no iota of chemicals in what you are applying on your body!! Secondly, you are cutting cost and saving up on a lot of money when you go homemade!

I remember the first homemade soap I made. After calculating all that I spent working on that soap, I realized that what I spent wasn't half of what I would have spent on my branded store bought soap!

In fact, I produced so much that lasted me for a long time! This was a feat that my store bought soap couldn't achieve!

Apart from that, making soaps by yourself gives you the liberty to be creative! You can decide to incorporate any type of ingredients (natural ingredients) that you want!

In summary, making your soap is amazing and interesting! A practice that will help you keep your skin nourished and healthy!

Now that you are well convinced that you have not made a mistake purchasing this book, let's flip the pages to our guest homemade soap – the lavender soap!!!

Chapter 1

Melt and Pour: Soap Recipes for Beginners

1 Grapefruit and Pink Himalayan Salt Soup

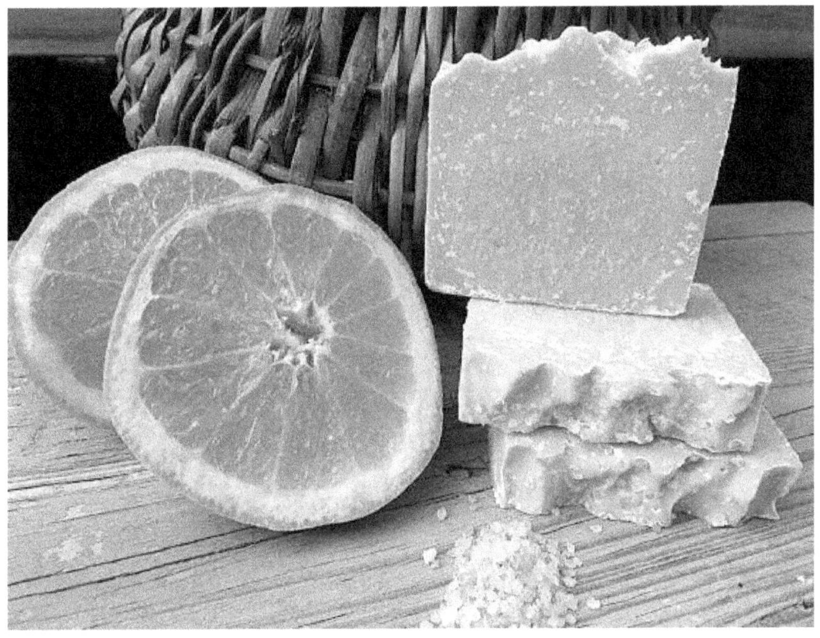

Serving: 6 to 12 soaps

Total Time: 6 minutes to make + 2 hours to harden

Ingredient list:

- 12 drops of grapefruit essential oil
- ¼ cup of pink Himalayan salt
- 1 pound of melt and pour soap base, goat's milk

Instruction:

a. Break the soap base up into a small 1-inch cube. Place in a glass bowl and melt in the microwave by cooking at 30 seconds increments, making sure to stir thoroughly after each time until the soap base has completely melted.

b. Mix in the pink Himalayan salt, followed by the grapefruit essential oil until well mixed with the melted soap base.

c. Transfer the mixture into the desired molds. Place the molds in a cool, dry location and let sit for 2 or more hours. Once hardened, pop the soap out of the molds and enjoy!

2 Avocado Soap

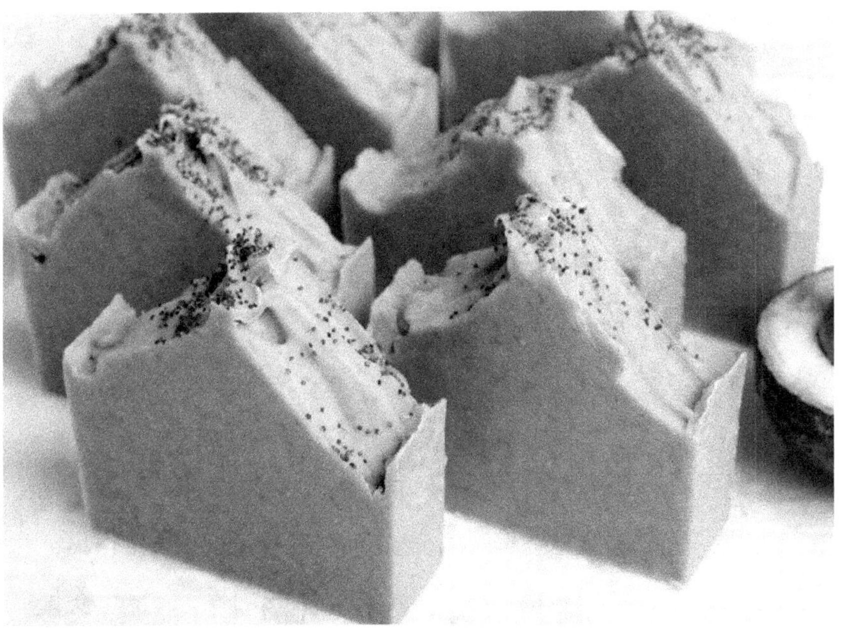

Serving: 6 to 10 soaps

Total Time: 10 minutes to make + 2 hours to harden

Ingredient list:

- 1/2 lemon
- 1 pound of melt and pour soap base
- 5 ounces of olive oil, extra-virgin
- 1 avocado

Instruction:

a. Cut the avocado in half and remove the seed, setting it to the side. Scoop out the pulp of the avocado and place in a blender. Blend until smooth.

b. Add the oil and the juice from half a lemon into the blender with the blended avocado and blend once again until smooth.

c. Chop the avocado seed into tiny pieces. Set to the side for the moment.

d. Break the soap base up into a small 1-inch cube. Place in a glass bowl and melt in the microwave by cooking at 30 seconds increments, making sure to stir thoroughly after each time until the soap base has completely melted.

e. Mix the avocado mixture from Step 2 and the chopped avocado seed from Step 3 into the melted soap base until well combined.

f. Transfer the mixture into the desired molds. Place the molds in a cool, dry location and let cool for 2 hours. Once set, pop the soap out of the molds and enjoy!

3 Earl Grey Tea Soap

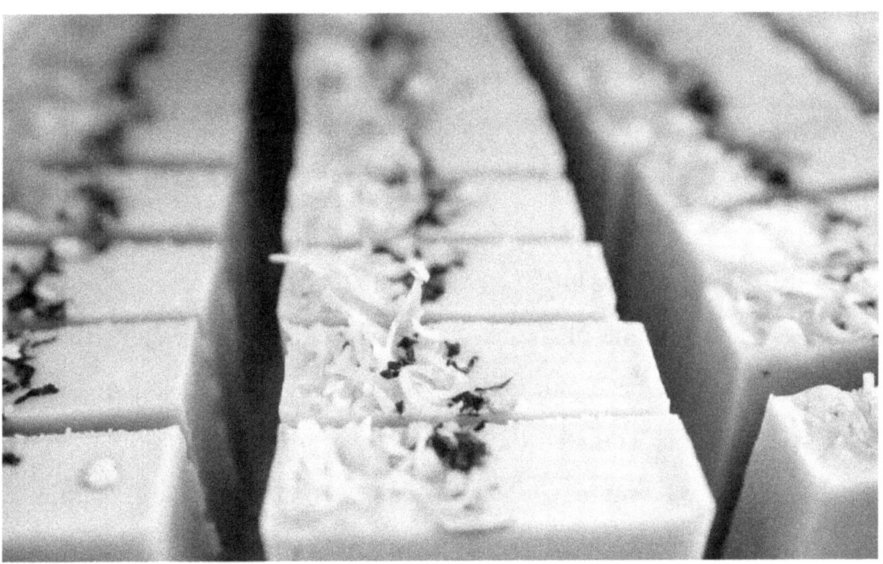

Serving: 6 to 12 soaps

Total Time: 10 minutes to make + several hours to harden

Ingredient list:

- ½ teaspoon of sweet orange essential oil

- 2 Earl Grey tea bags

- ½ teaspoon of litsea cubeba essential oil

- 2 pounds of melt and pour soap base

- 1 teaspoon of bergamot essential oil

Instruction:

a. Break the soap base up into a small 1-inch cube. Place in a glass bowl and melt in the microwave by cooking at 30 seconds increments, making sure to stir thoroughly after each time until the soap base has completely melted.

b. Mix in the essential oils until well combined. Open one of the tea bags and dump into the melted soap base. Stir until the dried tea is well distributed.

c. Transfer the mixture into the desired molds and immediately sprinkle the contents of the remaining tea bag over the top of the melted soap.

d. Place the molds in a cool, dry location and let cool for several hours. Once set, pop the soap out of the molds and enjoy!

4 Almond Honey and Chamomile Soap

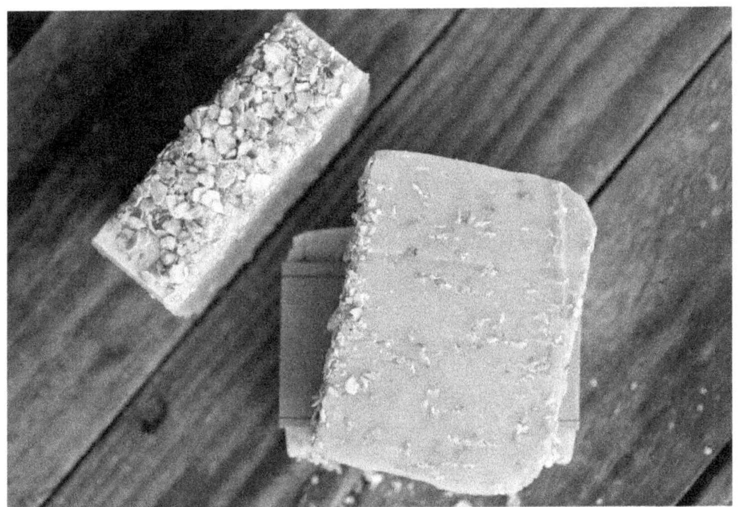

Serving: 12 to 18 soaps

Total Time: 10 minutes to make + several hours to harden

Ingredient list:

- 2 tablespoons of oatmeal, ground
- 3 chamomile tea bags
- 1 teaspoon of soap fragrance, honey almond
- 3 pounds of melt and pour base, goat's milk
- 2 tablespoons of honey

Instruction:

a. Break the melt and pour soap base into small pieces and place in a microwave-safe bowl. Heat in the microwave according to the soap base's directions. Make sure to stir the soap base periodically during the melting process.

b. Stir in the honey and ground oatmeal. Open the tea bags and dump the contents into the mixture, stirring until well combined.

c. Add the fragrance and stir for several seconds.

d. Pour the mixture into the desired molds. Let sit in a cool location until the soap is hardened, which should take a few hours, before using as needed.

5 Cilantro Lime Soap

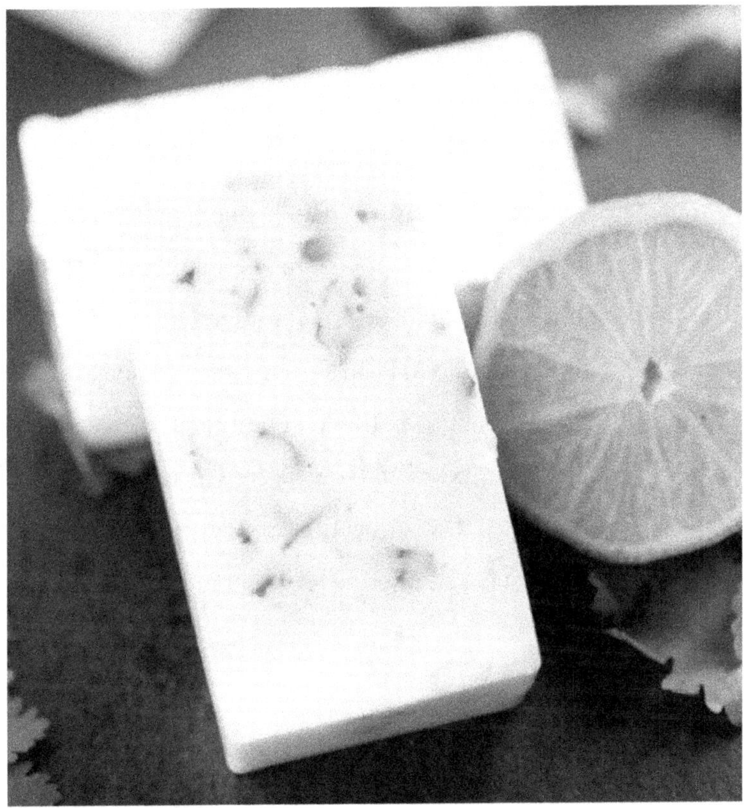

Serving: 6 to 12 soaps

Total Time: 5 minutes to make + 1 hour to set

Ingredient list:

- 20 drops of lime essential oil

- 16 cubes of melt and pour soap base, shea butter
- 3 tablespoons of cilantro, fresh and chopped

Instruction:

a. Place the melt and pour soap base into a glass bowl and melt in the microwave by cooking at 30 seconds increments, making sure to stir thoroughly after each time until the soap base has completely melted.

b. Stir the lime essential oil into the melted soap base. Fold in the cilantro until well combined.

c. Transfer the mixture into the desired molds. Place the molds in a cool, dry location and let cool for about an hour. Once set, pop the soap out of the molds and enjoy!

6 Coffee Soap

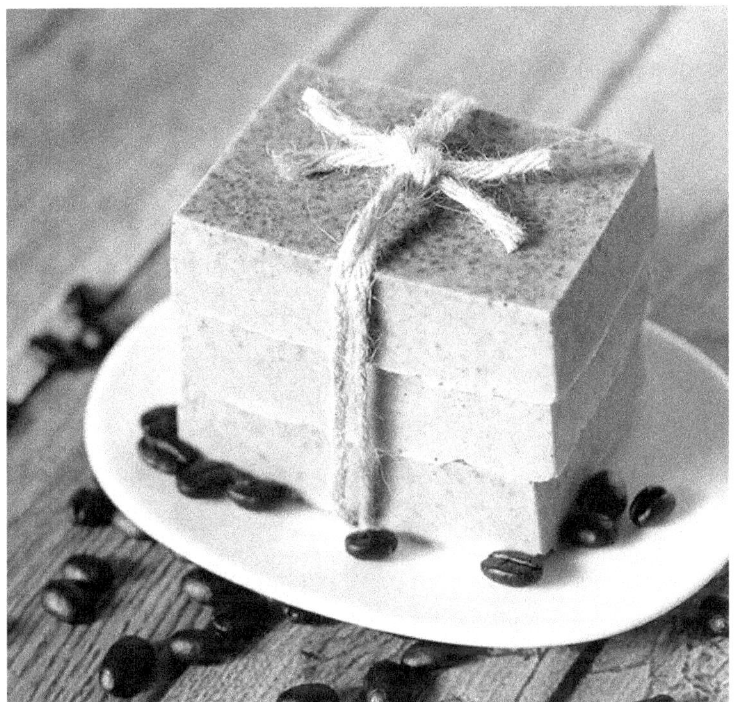

Serving: 6 to 12 soaps

Total Time: 10 minutes to make + 1 hour more hours to harden

Ingredient list:

- 1 tablespoon of coffee, ground
- 1 ½ pounds of melt and pour soap base, goat's milk

- 1 teaspoon of almond oil

- 1 ½ teaspoons of coffee soap fragrance oil

Instruction:

a. Cut the melt and pour soap base into small pieces and place in a microwave-safe bowl.

b. Heat in the microwave according to the soap base's directions. Make sure to stir the soap base periodically during the melting process.

c. Stir in the almond oil, coffee fragrance oil, and ground coffee until well combined.

d. Pour the melted soap mixture into the desired molds and let harden in a cool, dry location for an hour or more. Once the soap has hardened, remove them from the mold and use as needed.

7 Mint Cocoa Soap

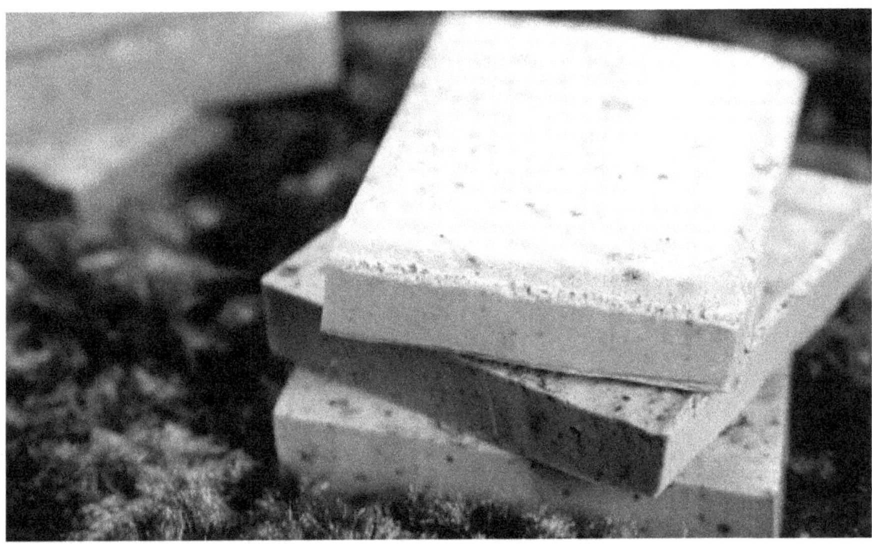

Serving: 6 to 12 soaps

Total Time: 6 minutes to make + 2 or more hours to set

Ingredient list:

- 10 drops of peppermint essential oil
- 2 tablespoons of fresh mint, chopped
- 1 pound melt and pour soap base, shea butter
- 2 tablespoons of cocoa powder, unsweetened

Instruction:

a. Break the soap base up into a small 1-inch cube. Place in a glass bowl and melt in the microwave by cooking at 30 seconds increments, making sure to stir thoroughly after each time until the soap base has completely melted.

b. Stir the peppermint essential oil into the melted soap base. Add the cocoa powder and stir until well combined. Mix in the chopped mint until it is evenly distributed throughout the mixture.

c. Transfer the mixture into the desired molds. Place the molds in a cool, dry location and let cool for 2 or more hours. Once set, pop the soap out of the molds and enjoy!

8 Cinnamon Oatmeal Soap

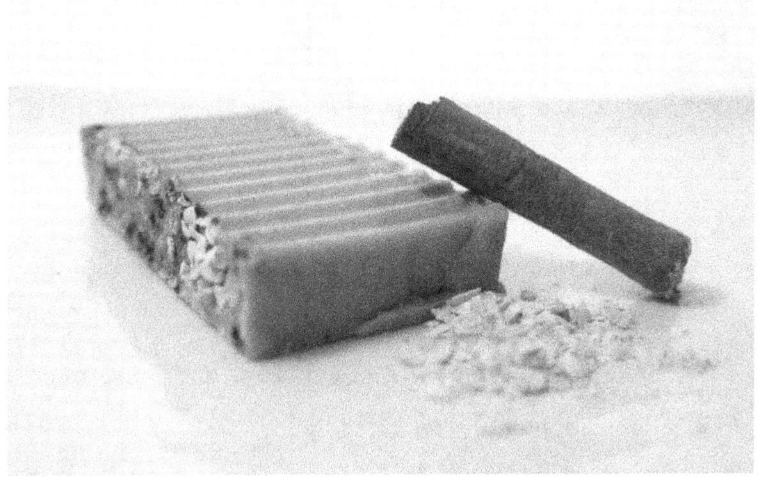

Serving: 6 to 12 soaps

Total Time: 5 to 10 minutes to make + 1 or more hours to set

Ingredient list:

- Oatmeal, for topping
- 8 ounces of melt and pour soap base
- ¼ teaspoon of ground cinnamon
- 1 drops of cinnamon essential oil

Instruction:

a. Cut the melt and pour soap into small cubes that are no bigger than 1-inch.

b. Microwave the melt and pour soap base in a microwave-safe container, making sure to follow the melting instructions located on the package. Make sure to periodically stir the soap base throughout the melting process to prevent burning.

c. Stir in the cinnamon essential oil and the ground cinnamon until well combined.

d. Pour the mixture into the molds. Sprinkle the oatmeal over the top of each soap and gently press the oatmeal into the melted soap.

e. Set the soap-filled mold in a cool, dry location and let harden for at least an hour. Once the soap is set, carefully pop them out of the mold and use as needed.

9 Lavender Soap

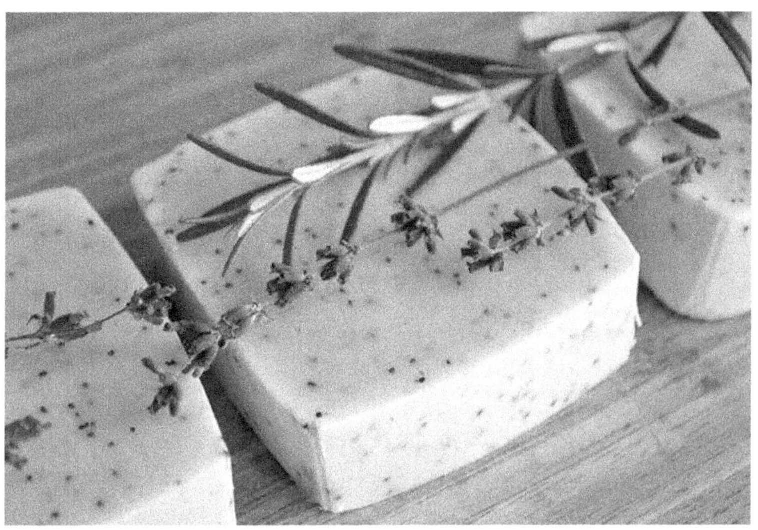

Serving: 12 soaps

Total Time: 20 minutes to make + 1 hour to harden

Ingredient list:

- 1 teaspoon of lavender essential oil
- 1 ½ tablespoons of lavender buds, dried
- 2 pounds melt and pour soap base, oatmeal

Instruction:

a. Cut the melt and pour soap into small cubes that are no bigger than 1-inch.

b. Microwave the melt and pour soap base in a microwave-safe container, making sure to follow the melting instructions located on the package. Make sure to periodically stir the soap base throughout the melting process to prevent burning.

c. Stir in the lavender essential oil, followed by the dried lavender buds. Once the two ingredients are well mixed in the melted soap base, continue with the remaining steps.

d. Pour the melted mixture into the silicone cupcake mold, filling each mold about half way full.

e. Set the molds in an area away from direct heat and sunlight, and let harden for about an hour. Once the soap is firm, pop them out of the molds and use as needed.

10 Lemon Soap

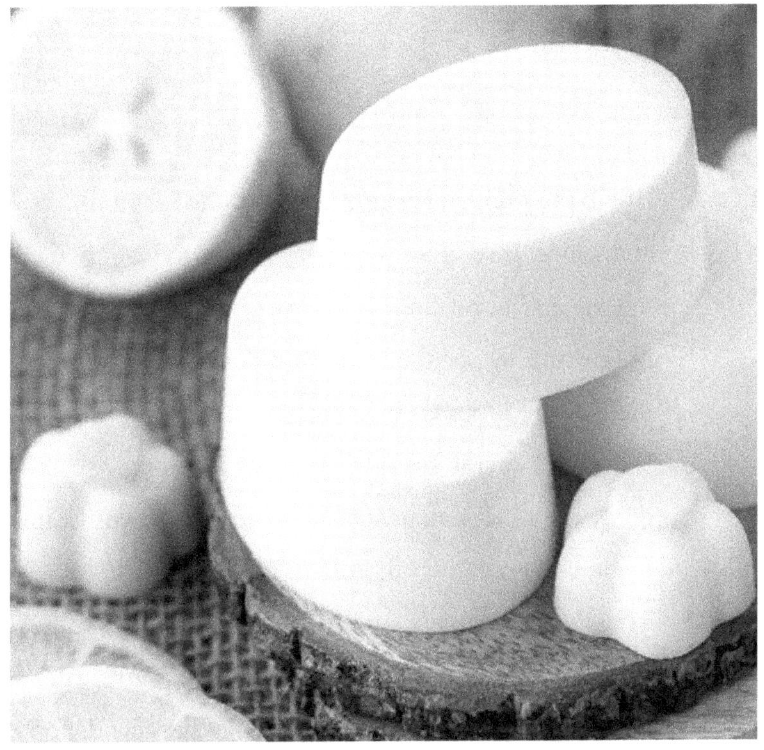

Serving: 6 to 12 soaps

Total Time: 5 to 10 minutes to make + 1 or more hours to harden

Ingredient list:

- Zest from 3 lemons, dried

- 1 ½ cups of melt and pour base, shea butter or <u>goat</u> milk

- 5 drops of lemon essential oil

Instruction:

a. Break the melt and pour soap base into small pieces and place in a microwave-safe bowl. Heat in the microwave according to the soap base's directions. Make sure to stir the soap base periodically during the melting process.

b. Wait for several seconds, but not too long as you don't want the soap to start to harden, and then stir in the lemon essential oil. Fold in the lemon zest.

c. Transfer the mixture into the desired molds. Set the molds in a cool, dry location and let the soap harden for an hour or more. Once the soap has hardened, pop them out of the molds and use as needed.

Chapter 2

Feminine and Floral Soap Recipes

11 Hollyhock Soap

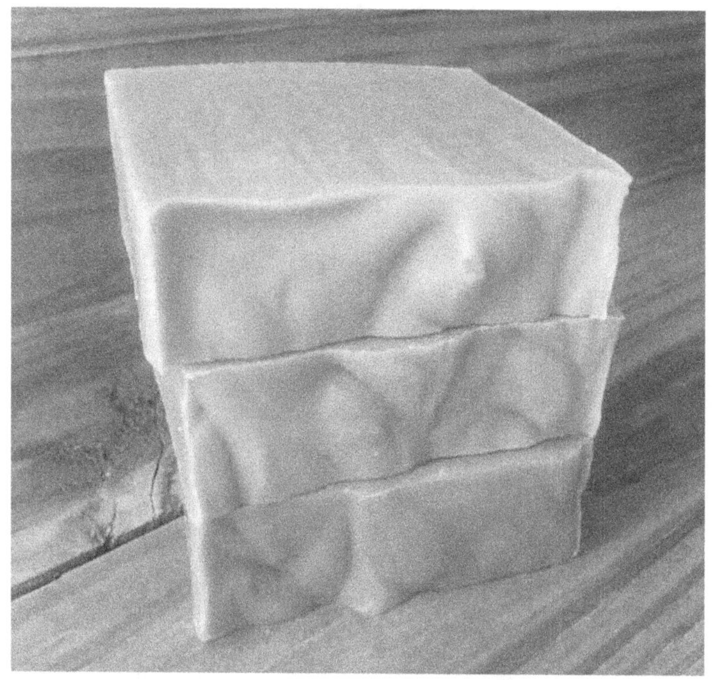

Serving: 6 to 12 soaps

Total Time: 20 to 25 minutes to make, 24 hours to set, 4 to 6 weeks to cure

Ingredient list:

- 2.5 ounces of castor oil
- 8 ounces of coconut oil

- 2.5 ounces of shea butter

- 1 teaspoon of rose clay

- 1 tablespoon of bergamot essential oil

- 4.13 ounces of lye

- 17 ounces of olive oil

- 10 ounces of hollyhock tea

Instruction:

a. Place the mint tea in a glass bowl. Slowly add the lye and stir until well combined. Set the bowl to the side.

b. In a double boiler, melt all the oils and mango butter together until well combined. Remove from heat and let cool for a minute or two before stirring in the essential oil.

c. Once the oil mixture and the lye mixture has cooled to a temperature of 90 to 110-degrees, pour the oil mixture into the lye mixture.

d. Using an immersion blender, blend the mixtures together until a trace forms. Stir in the red clay until well combined.

e. Pour the soap into the molds and cover. Let cool for about 24 hours. Pop the soaps out of the mold, cut and let cure in a well-ventilated area for 4 to 6 weeks.

12 Lemongrass and Coconut Soap

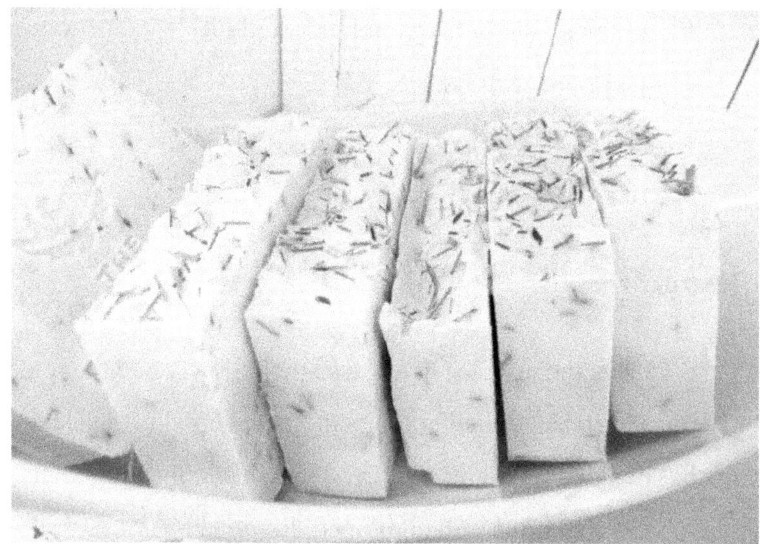

Serving: 8 to 12 soaps

Total Time: 25 to 35 minutes to make, 24 hours to harden, 3 to 6 weeks to cure

Ingredient list:

- 34 grams of lemongrass essential oil
- 2 ounces of castor oil
- 12 ounces of coconut oil
- 4.9 ounces sodium hydroxide
- 1 teaspoon of wheatgrass powder

- 8 grams of ginger essential oil
- 6 ounces of avocado oil
- 5 ounces of coconut milk
- 5 ounces of distilled water
- 6 ounces of shea butter
- 1 teaspoon of dried dill, cut
- 10 ounces of rice bran oil

Instruction:

a. Pour the distilled water into a glass bowl. Pour in the sodium hydroxide, doing so slowly to prevent splashing, and stir until well combined. Set the bowl to the side.

b. In a double boiler, melt all the oils and the shea butter while stirring constantly. Remove the mixture from heat once it is melted and well combined. Stir in the coconut milk.

c. Once the oil mixture has cooled to a temperature between 100 and 115 degrees, pour it carefully into the sodium hydroxide mixture. Use a stick blender to blend to an emulsified state. Stir in the essential oils until well combined.

d. Remove about ¼ of the soap mixture and place in a
   container. Add the wheatgrass powder and stir until
   well combined.

e. Stir the dried dill into the remaining soap mixture to
   give it a nice yellow color.

f. Pour about half of the dill-colored mixture into the
   desired mold. Drizzle the wheat grass-colored
   mixture over the top, covering with the remaining
   dill-colored mixture.

g. Cover the molds and let cool for about 24 hours. Pop
   the soaps out of the mold, cut and let cure in a well-
   ventilated area for 3 to 6 weeks.

13 Herbal Mint Soap

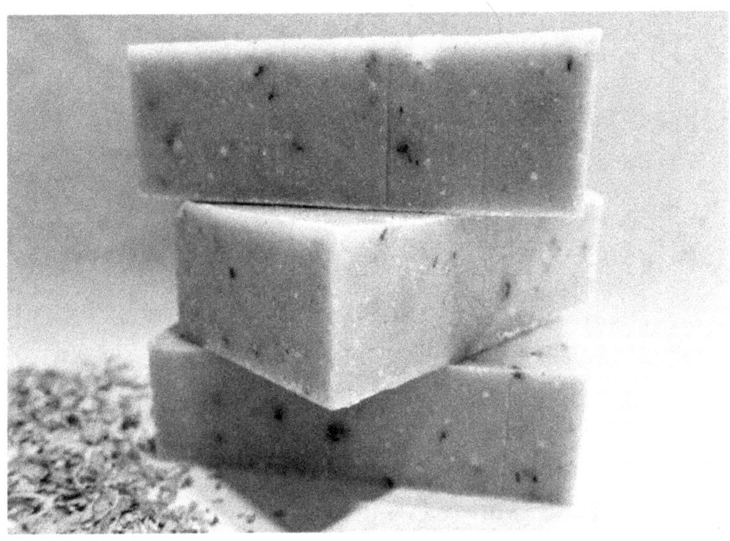

Serving:

Total Time: 30 to 35 minutes, 24 hours to set, 4 to 6 weeks to cure

Ingredient list:

- 4 ounces of avocado oil
- 4 ounces of castor oil
- 24 ounces of coconut oil
- 9 ounces of lye
- 19 ounces of mint tea, cooled

- 2 ½ tablespoons of peppermint essential oil
- 1 ½ tablespoons of French green clay mixed with 3 tablespoons water
- 2 ounces of mango butter
- 28 ounces of olive oil

Instruction:

- Place the mint tea in a glass bowl. Slowly add the lye and stir until well combined. Set the bowl to the side.
- In a double boiler, melt all the oils and mango butter together until well combined. Remove from heat and let cool for a minute or two before stirring in the essential oil.
- Once the oil mixture and the lye mixture has cooled to a temperature of 90 to 110-degrees, pour the oil mixture into the lye mixture.
- Using an immersion blender, blend the mixtures together until a trace forms. Stir in the green clay/water mixture until well combined.
- Pour the soap into the molds and cover. Let cool for about 24 hours. Pop the soaps out of the mold, cut and let cure in a well-ventilated area for 4 to 6 weeks.

Chapter 3

Masculine-Inspired Soap Recipes

14 Cucumber Soap

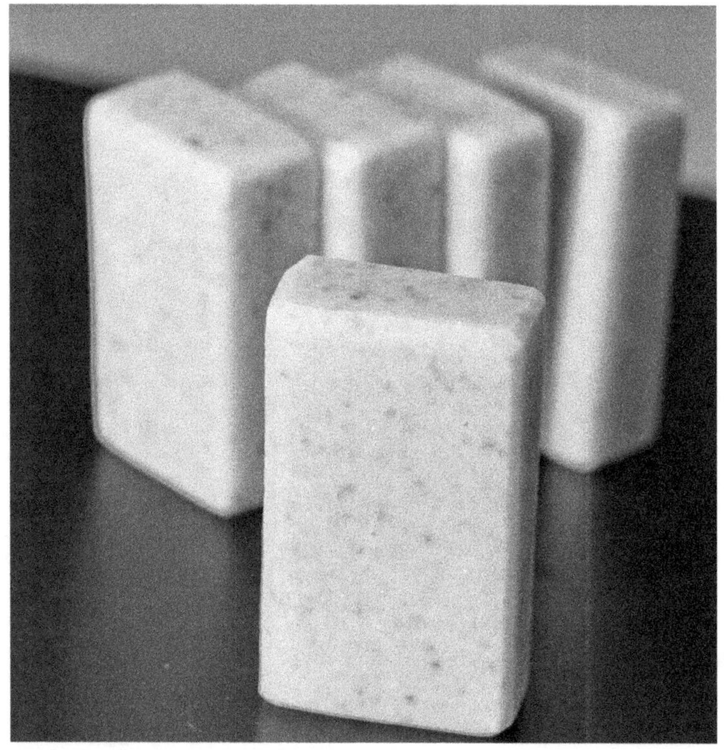

Serving: 6 to 10 soaps

Total Time: 35 minutes to make, 24 hours to set, 4 to 6 weeks to cure

Ingredient list:

- 3 ounces of cucumber, unpeeled

- 2 ounces of avocado oil

- 2 ounces of shea butter

- 4 ounces of rice bran oil

- 8 ounces of coconut oil

- 3.83 ounces of lye

- 9 ounces of water, distilled and chilled

- ½ tablespoon of French green clay + 1 tablespoon water

Instruction:

a. Place the water and the cucumber into a food processor and puree for several seconds. Strain the cucumber pulp from the mixture and discard. Pour the cucumber juice into a glass bowl.

b. Slowly add the lye to the cucumber juice and stir until well combined. Set the bowl to the side.

c. In a double boiler, melt all the oil and butter together until well combined. Remove from heat.

d. Once the oil mixture and the lye mixture has cooled to a temperature of 90 to 110-degrees, pour the oil mixture into the lye mixture.

e. Using an immersion blender, blend the mixtures together until a trace forms. Stir in the green clay/water mixture until well combined.

f.   Pour the soap into the molds and cover. Let cool for
     about 24 hours. Pop the soaps out of the mold, cut
     and let cure in a well-ventilated area for 4 to 6 weeks.

15 Vanilla Bean and Bourbon Whiskey Soap

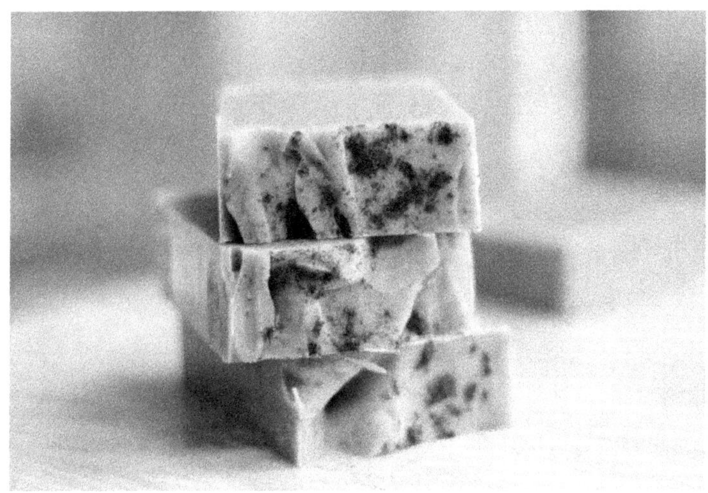

Serving: 10 to 12 soaps

Total Time: 30 minutes to make, 24 hours to set, 4 to 6 weeks to cure

Ingredient list:

- 2.5 ounces of avocado oil
- 9 ounces of distilled water
- 1 ounce of bourbon
- 12.5 ounces of coconut oil

- 2 ounces of sunflower oil
- 1 ounce of grapefruit essential oil
- 2 ounces of shea butter
- 2 tablespoons of vanilla bean powder
- 4.8 ounces of sodium hydroxide
- .5 ounces of ylang ylang essential oil
- .5 ounces of almond essential oil
- 15 ounces of olive oil
- .5 ounces of juniper essential oil

Instruction:

a. Pour the distilled water into a glass bowl, slowly adding the sodium hydroxide, and stir until well combined. Set the bowl to the side.

b. In a double boiler, melt all the oils and the shea butter while stirring constantly. Remove the mixture from heat and let cool for a minute or two. Stir in the essential oils, followed by the vanilla bean powder.

c. Once the oil mixture has cooled to about 90-degrees, pour it carefully into the sodium hydroxide mixture. Use a stick blender to blend to an emulsified state.

d. Stir in the bourbon until well combined and immediately pour into the desired molds. If desired, sprinkle some of the vanilla bean powder over the top.

e. Cover the molds and let cool for about 24 hours. Pop the soaps out of the mold, cut and let cure in a well-ventilated area for 4 to 6 weeks.

Chapter 4

Simple Seasonal Soap Recipes

16 Peppermint Soap

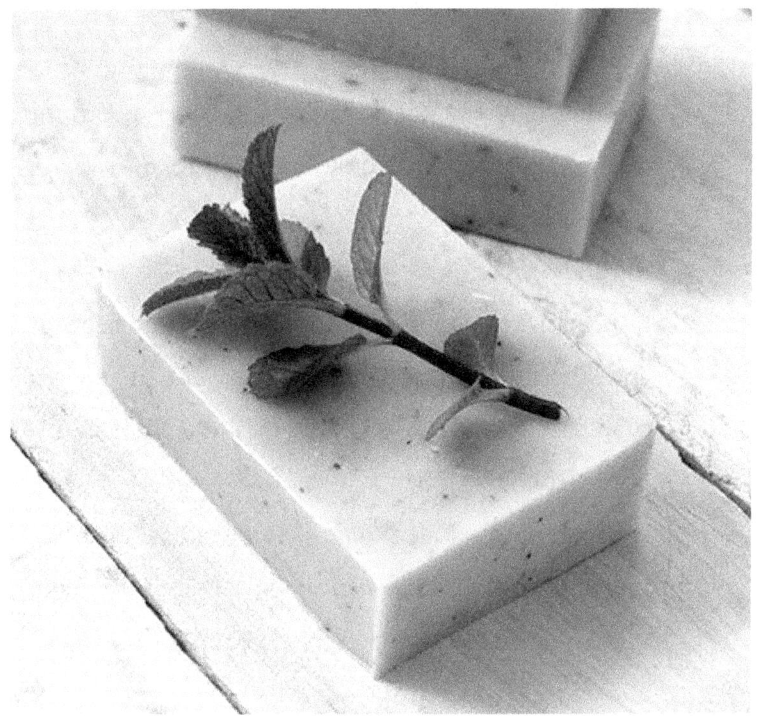

Serving: 8 to 12 soaps

Total Time: 8 minutes to make + 45 minutes to harden

Ingredient list:

- 44 drops of peppermint essential oil

- 1 ounce of red jojoba beads

- 2 pounds of melt and pour soap base, goat's milk

Instruction:

a. Break the soap base up into a small 1-inch cube. Place in a glass bowl and melt in the microwave by cooking at 30 seconds increments, making sure to stir thoroughly after each time until the soap base has completely melted.

b. Stir the peppermint essential oil into the melted soap base until well combined. Add in the red jojoba beads and stir until well distributed. Make sure the melted soap base is below 130 degrees to prevent the jojoba beads from dissolving.

c. Transfer the mixture into the desired molds. Place the molds in a cool, dry location and let cool for about 45 minutes. Once set, pop the soap out of the molds and enjoy!

17 Cranberry Vanilla Soap

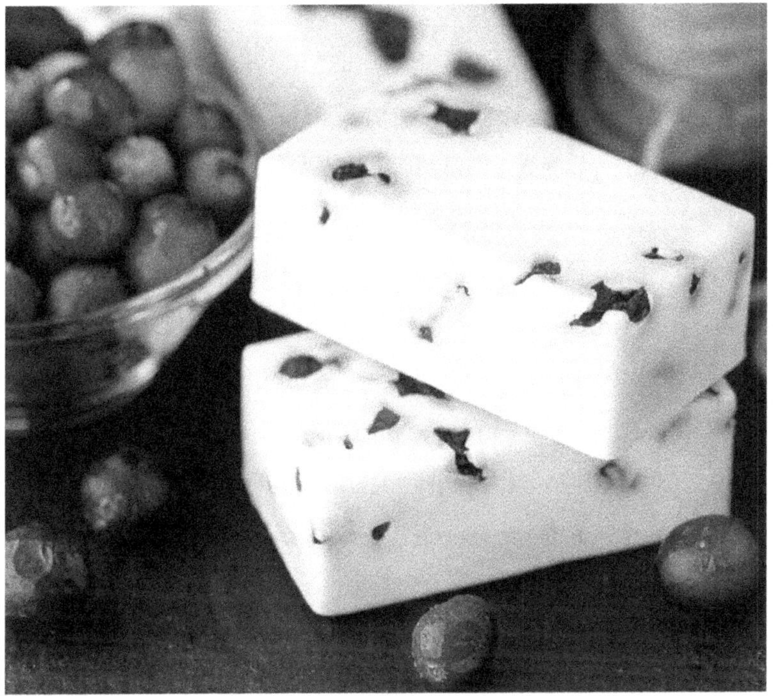

Serving: 6 to 12 soaps

Total Time: 5 minutes to make + 1 hour to harden

Ingredient list:

- ¼ cup of cranberries, dried

- 20 drops of soap fragrance, vanilla

- 1 pound of melt and pour soap base, shea butter

Instruction:

a. Line the bottom of the soap mold with the cranberries. Set to the side for the moment.

b. Cut the soap base up into small 1-inch cubed. Place in a glass bowl and melt in the microwave by cooking at 30 seconds increments, making sure to stir thoroughly after each time until the soap base has completely melted.

c. Mix in the vanilla fragrance until well combined.

d. Transfer the mixture into the desired molds. Place the molds in a cool, dry location and let cool for an hour or until set. Once set, pop the soap out of the molds

18 Pumpkin Pie Spice Soap

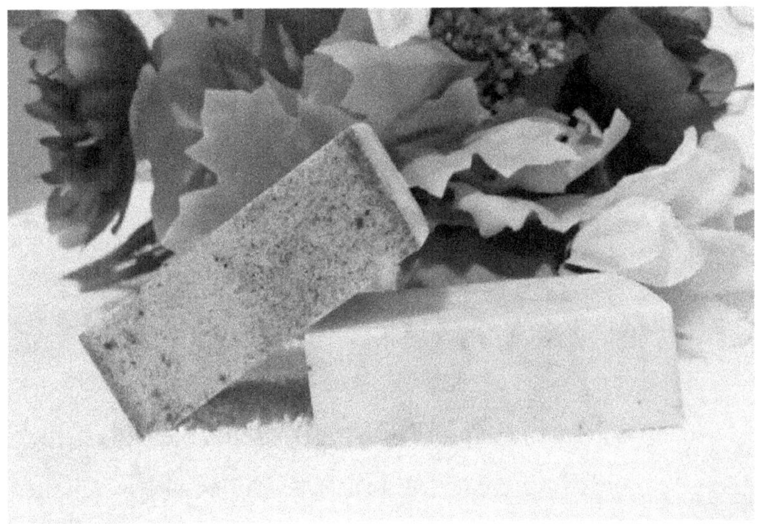

Serving: 8 bars of soap

Total Time: 10 minutes to make + 30 minutes to 1 hour to set

Ingredient list:

- 2 drops of red soap colorant
- 4 drops of yellow soap colorant
- 2 tablespoons of pumpkin pie spice
- 2 pounds of melt and pour soap base, shea butter

Instruction:

a. Break the soap base up into a small 1-inch cube. Place in a glass bowl and melt in the microwave by cooking at 30 seconds increments, making sure to stir thoroughly after each time until the soap base has completely melted.

b. Add the pumpkin pie spice to the melted soap base and stir until well combined. Stir in the colorant to get a nice pumpkin-ish shade.

c. Transfer the mixture into the desired molds. Place the molds in a cool, dry location and let cool for about 30 minutes to an hour. Once set, pop the soap out of the molds and enjoy!

19 Spiced Apple Soap

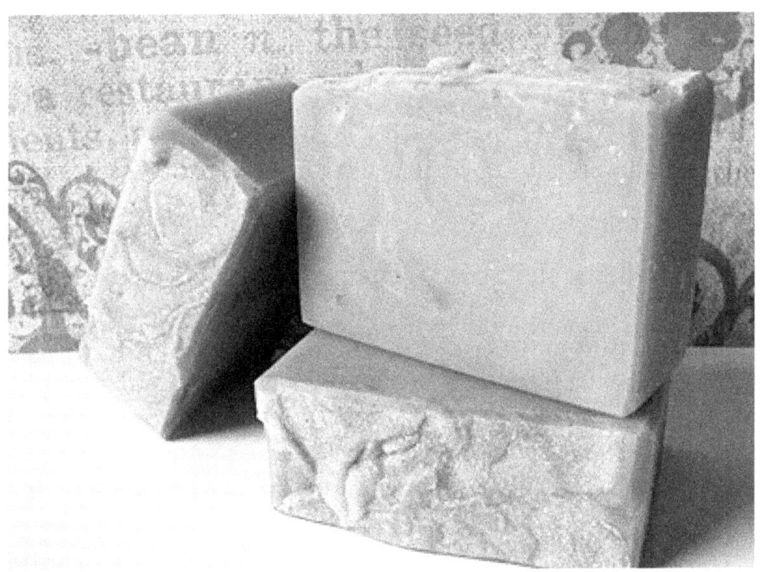

Serving: 4 to 8 soaps

Total Time: 5 minutes to make + 1 to 2 hours to harden

Ingredient list:

- ½ teaspoon of apple pie spice
- 2 to 3 drops of orange soap colorant
- 1 pound of melt and pour soap base, goat's milk
- ¼ ounce of apple soap fragrance

Instruction:

a. Cut the soap base up into small 1-inch cubed. Place in a glass bowl and melt in the microwave by cooking at 30 seconds increments, making sure to stir thoroughly after each time until the soap base has completely melted.

b. Stir the apple soap fragrance into the melted mixture, followed by the soap colorant. You can add more or less fragrance and colorant to get the desired scent and coloring.

c. Fold the apple pie spice into the mixture until well combined.

d. Transfer the mixture into the desired molds. Place the molds in a cool, dry location and let cool for an hour or until set. Once set, pop the soap out of the molds and enjoy!

20 Happy Fall Y'All Soap

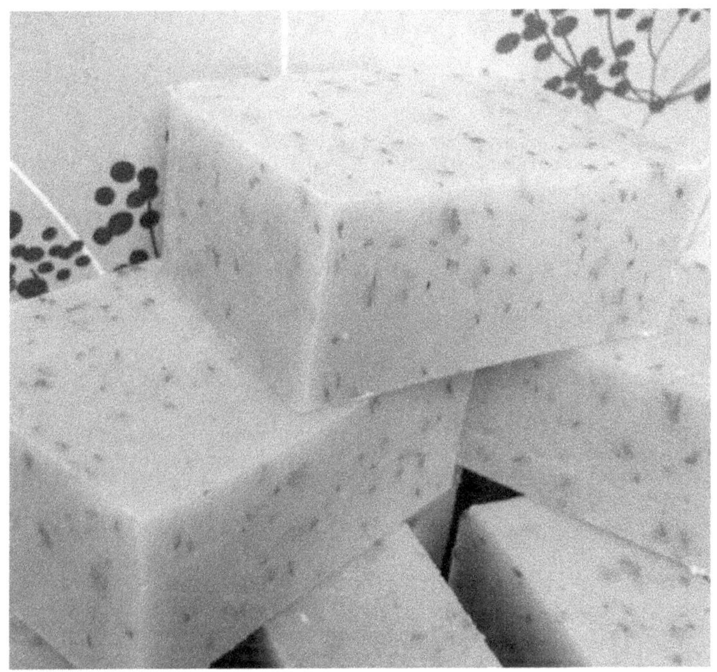

Serving: 8 to 12 soaps

Total Time: 8 minutes to make + a few hours to set

Ingredient list:

- 20 drops of cinnamon leaf essential oil

- 20 drops of clove bud essential oil

- 40 drops of sweet Orange essential oil

- ¼ cup of walnut shells, ground

- 2 pounds of melt and pour soap base

Instruction:

a. Break the soap base up into a small 1-inch cube. Place in a glass bowl and melt in the microwave by cooking at 30 seconds increments, making sure to stir thoroughly after each time until the soap base has completely melted.

b. Add the ground walnut shells to the melted soap base and stir until well combined. Stir in all three of the essential oils until well mixed.

c. Transfer the mixture into the desired molds. Place the molds in a cool, dry location and let cool for a few hours. Once set, pop the soap out of the molds and enjoy!

Chapter 5

Skin Condition-Friendly Soap Recipes

21 Calamine Soap

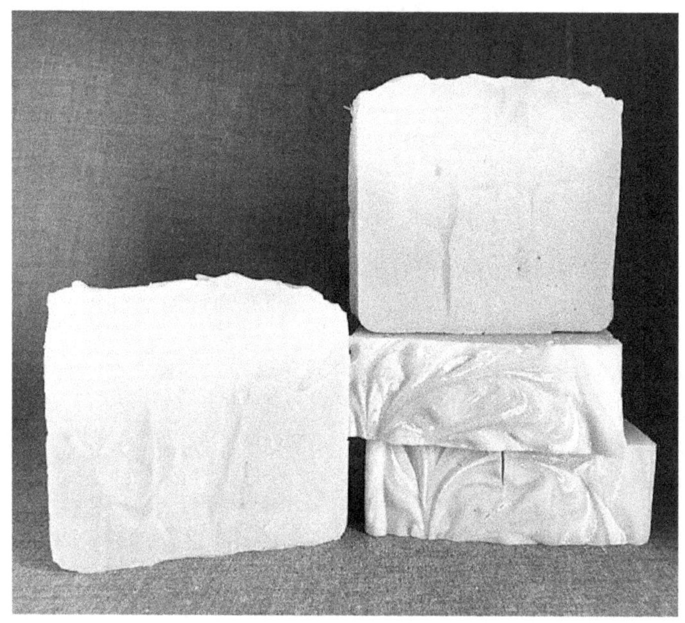

Serving: 8 to 14 soaps

Total Time: 30 minutes to make, 24 hours to harden, 4 to 6 weeks to cure

Ingredient list:

- .4 ounces of shea butter
- ½ tablespoon of red oxide
- 1 pound 6 ounces of soybean oil

- .8 ounces of cocoa butter
- 2 pounds of olive oil
- 1 ounce tea tree essential oil
- 1.5 ounces of lavender essential oil
- ½ cup of zinc oxide
- 38 ounces of water
- 1 pound 2 ounces palm oil
- 2 pounds of coconut oil
- 15 ounces of lye
- 1.5 ounces of chamomile essential oil

Instruction:

a. Place the water in a glass bowl. Slowly add the lye and stir until well combined. Set the bowl to the side.

b. In a double boiler, melt all the oil, except the essential oils, and butter together until well combined. Remove from heat.

c. Once the oil mixture and the lye mixture has cooled to a temperature of 100 and 125-degrees, pour the oil mixture into the lye mixture. Add the red oxide and the zinc oxide.

d. Using an immersion blender, blend the mixtures together until a trace forms. At the trace, stir in the essential oils.

e. Pour the soap into the molds and cover. Let cool for about 24 hours. Pop the soaps out of the mold, cut and let cure in a well-ventilated area for 4 to 6 weeks.

22 Bamboo-Charcoal Soap

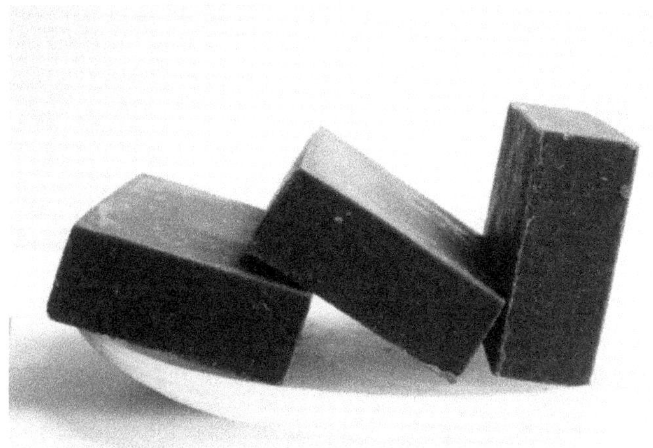

Serving: 8 to 12 soaps

Total Time: 20 minutes to make, 24 hours to harden, 4 to 6 weeks to cure

Ingredient list:

- 1.6 ounces castor oil
- 4.7 ounces of lye
- 8 ounces olive oil
- 1 tablespoon of bamboo charcoal powder
- 8 ounces of coconut oil

- 12.1 ounces of water, distilled

- 4.8 ounces of palm kernel oil

- 9.6 ounces palm oil

Instruction:

a. Pour the distilled water into a glass bowl. Slowly add the lye and stir until well combined. Set the bowl to the side.

b. In a double boiler, melt all the oils together until well combined. Remove from heat and let cool for a minute or two before whisking in the bamboo charcoal powder.

c. Once the oil mixture and the lye mixture has cooled to a temperature of 90 to 110-degrees, pour the oil mixture into the lye mixture.

d. Use an immersion blender to blend the mixtures until a trace forms.

e. Pour the soap into the molds and cover. Let cool for about 24 hours. Pop the soaps out of the mold, cut and let cure in a well-ventilated area for 4 to 6 weeks.

23 Aloe Vera Soap

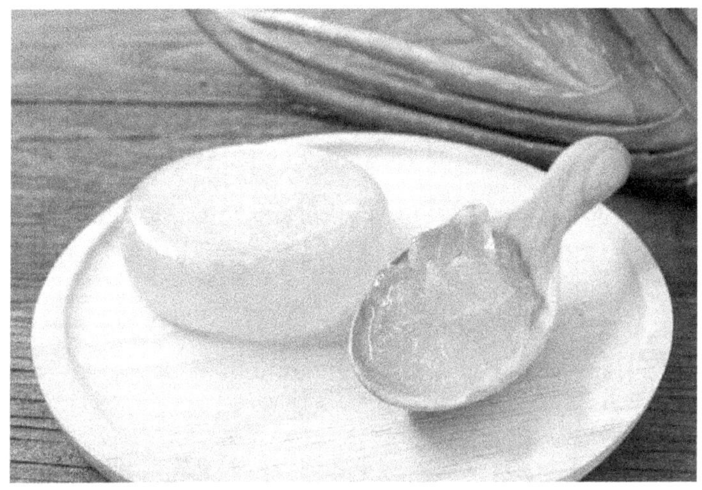

Serving: 8 to 12 soaps

Total Time: 25 to 30 minutes to make, 24 hours to set, 4 to 6 weeks to cure

Ingredient list:

- 13.4 ounces of olive oil
- 14.9 ounces of coconut oil
- 2.5 ounces of shea butter
- 10.5 ounces of lard
- 9.6 ounces of aloe gel

- 9.9 ounces of water, distilled
- 6.7ounces of lye

Instruction:

a. Pour the distilled water into a glass bowl, slowly adding the sodium hydroxide, and stir until well combined. Set the bowl to the side.
b. In a double boiler, melt all the oils, the butter, and the lard together until well combined. Remove from heat.
c. Once the oil mixture and the lye mixture has cooled to a temperature of 120 to 130-degrees, pour the oil mixture into the lye mixture. Stir in the aloe vera gel.
d. Using a stick blender, blend the mixtures together until a trace forms.
e. Cover the molds and let cool for about 24 hours. Pop the soaps out of the mold, cut and let cure in a well-ventilated area for 4 to 6 weeks.

24 Tea Tree Oil Soap

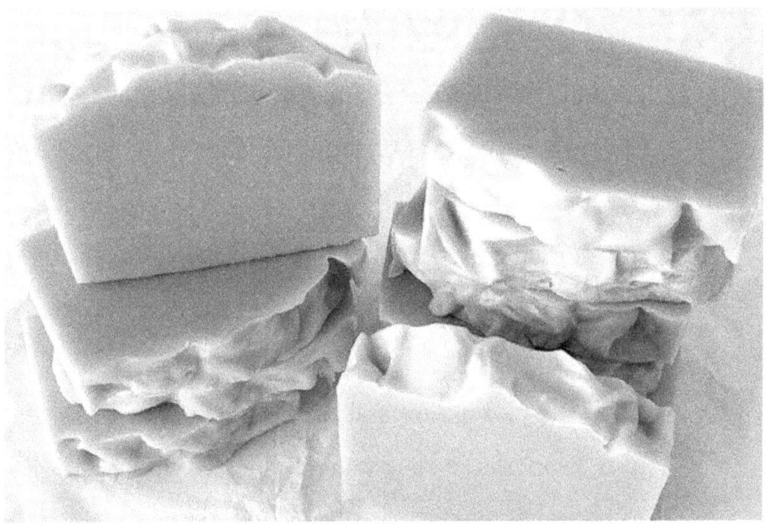

Serving: 8 to 12 soaps

Total Time: 25 to 30 minutes, 24 hours to harden, 4 to 6 weeks to cure

Ingredient list:

- 7.2 ounces of olive oil
- 2.27 ounces of lye
- 2.08 ounces of sweet almond oil
- 1.92 ounces of avocado oil
- 6.08 ounces of water, distilled
- 0.7 ounces of tea tree oil

- 4.8 ounces of coconut oil

Instruction:

a. Pour the distilled water into a glass bowl. Slowly add the lye and stir until well combined. Set the bowl to the side.

b. In a double boiler, melt all the oils, except for the tea tree oil, together until well combined. Remove from heat.

c. Once the oil mixture and the lye mixture has cooled to a temperature of about 95-degrees, pour the oil mixture into the lye mixture.

d. Use an immersion blender to blend the mixtures until a trace forms. At trace, mix in the tea tree oil.

e. Pour the soap into the molds and cover. Let cool for about 24 hours. Pop the soaps out of the mold, cut and let cure in a well-ventilated area for 4 to 6 weeks.

25 Pine Tar Soap

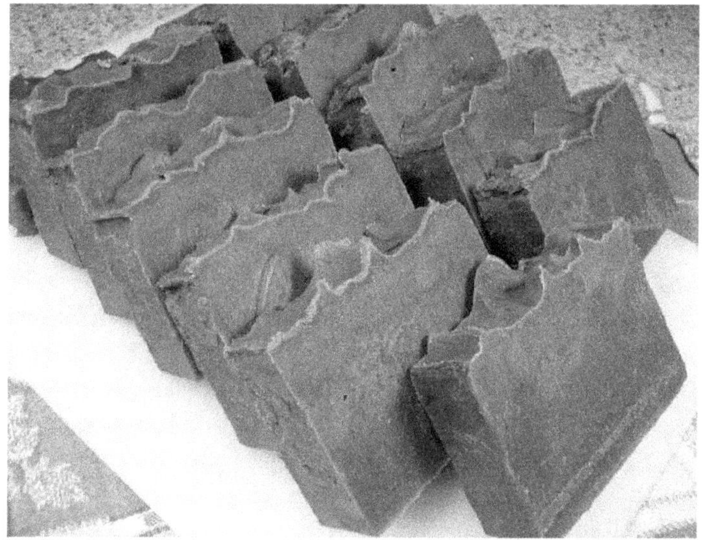

Serving: 4 bars

Total Time: 20 to 25 minutes to make, 24 hours to harden, 4 to 6 weeks to cure

Ingredient list:

- 3.9 ounces of water, distilled
- 7 ounces of olive oil
- 1.45 ounces of lye
- 1 teaspoon of sodium lactate

- .6 ounces of castor oil

- .15 ounces of eucalyptus essential oil

- 2.6 ounces of coconut oil

- 1.8 ounces of pine tar

Instruction:

a. Place the distilled water in a glass bowl. Slowly add the lye and stir until well combined. Stir in the sodium lactate. Set the bowl to the side.

b. In a double boiler, melt the coconut, olive, and castor oil and the pine tar together until well combined. Remove from heat and let cool for a minute or two before stirring in the essential oil.

c. Once the oil mixture and the lye mixture has cooled to a temperature of about 80-degrees, pour the oil mixture into the lye mixture.

d. Using an immersion blender, blend the mixtures together until a trace forms.

e. Pour the soap into the molds and cover. Let cool for about 24 hours. Pop the soaps out of the mold, cut and let cure in a well-ventilated area for 4 to 6 weeks.